Glucose Transformation:

Dealing with your blood sugar to transform your life

Charlott J. Leon

Table of content

INTRODUCTION

The road to health may have its share of obstacles, particularly regarding managing sugar levels. Blood sugar levels are nothing to laugh at; either too high or too low might have negative consequences. Because of this, many individuals are searching for natural ways to maintain healthy blood sugar levels.

When blood glucose levels are higher than what our cells can utilize, the hormone insulin is produced to remove the excess glucose from circulation and store it as fat for potential use later.

This precisely calibrated device performs well when blood glucose levels are mostly steady.

However, how we now consume, which includes mindless nibbling on highly processed and sugary foods, may result in sharp spikes in blood sugar that can harm the body and the brain.

Large amounts of insulin are then released, which might have similar negative effects.

Weight reduction is difficult since insulin turns the path to our fat cells into a one-way street. However, if our insulin levels and, by extension, our blood glucose levels are stable, we lose weight.

Canadian researchers found that an insulin drop usually follows weight reduction in a study of 5,600 participants conducted in 2021.

Numerous studies have shown that recurrent glucose spikes may impact various factors, including our immune system's health and risk of heart disease, as well as our mood, sleep, weight, and skin.

You can experience hunger, cravings, exhaustion, more severe menopausal symptoms, migraines, restless nights, and cognitive fog in the short term.

See-sawing glucose levels over time contribute to aging and the onset of diseases, including Alzheimer's disease, cancer, type 2 diabetes, fatty liver disease, acne, eczema, psoriasis, and arthritis.

Hormonal abnormalities brought on by glucose surges may severely affect libido. You can understand why maintaining consistent glucose levels and avoiding spikes might significantly enhance your sex life when you consider that glucose highs and lows can cause a lack of energy, poor sleep, and negative emotions.

Other variables also influence the glucose curves. Everyone's meal can cause radically diverse blood glucose reactions in various individuals; the rate at which you turn that meal into glucose and how quickly your body reacts to elevated glucose levels may be influenced by your natural baseline insulin levels.

Your muscle mass (the more muscles you have to pull glucose out of your circulation) and the populations of gut microorganisms may impact this (some guts break down food or release chemical messengers more effectively).

It also relies on your level of fatigue or stress (both may cause the production of stress hormones that alter metabolism), your level of hydration or dehydration, whether you were active, and how well or poorly you slept. Studies have also shown that when you anticipate eating something sweet, your body proactively sets off many chemical cascades, which might result in a greater increase than if you weren't anticipating being served a biscuit.

I'll share my tips for altering your eating habits to flatten the curve in this book. You'll not only feel better but also lose weight as your body becomes more adept at functioning.

CHAPTER 1

WHAT IS GLUCOSE

The term "sugar" refers to various caloric sweeteners in various sorts and forms. Table sugar is the most widely used kind of sugar. According to science, table sugar is sucrose and a disaccharide made up of an equal mixture of fructose and glucose, two monosaccharides.

Monosaccharides, isolated sugar molecules, are often called "simple" sugars. Fructose, galactose, and glucose are the three primary monosaccharides humans eat. The three types of disaccharides (two connected sugar units) most important for human nutrition are lactose, maltose, and sucrose, which combine in various combinations. The link between all of them is glucose. It is a component of maltose, made up of two connected glucose units, lactose, which is linked with galactose, and sucrose, which is linked with fructose.

In addition to being essential to disaccharides, glucose is also necessary for life. Our body uses glucose primarily for energy, and certain tissues, including the brain, need a steady supply. Since glucose flows in our circulation as a readily accessible energy source, it is called "blood sugar." Additionally, the body stores it as glycogen to be used as an energy source when the blood supply of glucose may be insufficient.

What Is The Source Of Glucose?

The most prevalent monosaccharide in nature is glucose. It is produced by photosynthesis in plants. Chains of linked glucose are stored by certain plants. Starch is the name for these chains. Foods that often include starch include maize, potatoes, rice, and wheat. From these entire food sources, starch is professionally separated to create glucose, maltodextrins, polyols, dextrose, and high fructose corn syrup, which are then utilized as components in the creation of a variety of meals, drinks, dressings, and sauces.

Some foods naturally include glucose monosaccharides but not as part of the starch component. Honey is the entire food with the highest concentration of glucose monosaccharides, followed by dates, apricots, raisins, currants, cranberries, prunes, and figs.

Why Is Glucose So Important?

The body uses glucose as its primary energy source. You get it mostly from the carbs you consume, such as sugar and wheat. Your body's cells take it up via the blood and utilize it as fuel.

Blood sugar or blood glucose refers to the quantity of glucose in your blood. Insulin, a hormone that transports glucose from the circulation and into cells where it may be utilized as fuel, helps your body control blood sugar levels.

If this procedure is disturbed, issues could arise. For instance, with diabetes, your body either produces insufficient insulin or fails to utilize it properly, which results in hyperglycemia or high blood sugar. Hypoglycemia, or low blood sugar, may also happen. Serious health issues may result from both high and low blood sugar levels.

Can The Body Produce Glucose?

Glucose is necessary for our bodies to operate. Given that our brain consumes roughly 60% of the glucose that our bodies consume, it is very important for this organ. But glucose doesn't necessarily have to come from food and drink right away. The body produces its own glucose to make sure we always have plenty. By dissolving glycogen to release the glucose, it contains, this may be accomplished. Between meals or during times of vigorous exercise, glycogen is broken down. The process of gluconeogenesis, which is mostly carried out by the liver, allows the body to create glucose from non-carbohydrate sources. When glucose production is too low or nonexistent, and glycogen reserves are depleted, as happens during extended fasting or famine, gluconeogenesis takes place.

What Do Plants Do To Make Glucose?

The most prevalent monosaccharide in nature is glucose. It is produced by photosynthesis in plants. Chains of linked glucose are stored by certain plants. Starch is the name for these chains. Foods that often include starch include maize, potatoes, rice, and wheat. From these entire food sources, starch is professionally separated to create dextrose, glucose, polyols, maltodextrins, and high fructose corn syrup, which are then utilized as components in the creation of a variety of meals, drinks, dressings, and sauces.

Some foods naturally include glucose monosaccharides but not as part of the starch component. Honey is the entire food with the highest concentration of glucose monosaccharides, followed by dates, apricots, raisins, currants, cranberries, prunes, and figs.

Depending on where it comes from, the sugar we eat is either referred to as natural sugar or added sugar. If glucose is taken straight from whole foods like apricots and dates, it is regarded as a natural sugar. When ingested from packaged foods and drinks to which it has been added during manufacture, glucose is regarded as an added sugar. Sadly, just approximately one in ten persons in America consume the recommended daily amounts of fruits and vegetables, while six out of ten consume more added sugars than is healthy.

How Glucose Gets Into The Bloodstream

Starches and simple sugars are both types of carbohydrates that include the molecule glucose, generally known as blood sugar. Because it is the brain's main source of energy and a substantial source of energy for all body cells, glucose is a crucial biological chemical. Glucose is transported from the digestive tract to the body's cells with the assistance of the circulatory system.

Giving cells energy is the biomolecule glucose's main purpose. The glucose present in the blood is taken up by body cells, where it is chemically burned to produce energy molecules that are used to carry out cellular operations. Some cells, including those in the muscles and liver, store glucose and release it while you're fasting. The most widespread of the carbohydrate molecules is often said to be glucose.

Several cell membranes must be crossed for glucose to go from the digestive system, where it is found after a meal, into the body cells, where it is used. Since cell membranes are composed of fatty substances and glucose is water soluble, glucose cannot independently traverse cell membranes. Transporter molecules must instead transfer it into and out of cells. However, glucose does dissolve quickly in circulation.

After being absorbed from the gut, glucose initially enters the circulation. Dedicated cellular transporters, known as sodium-dependent hexose transporters, move glucose across intestinal epithelial cells. Once glucose has passed through the intestinal lining, it may disintegrate in the blood and circulate throughout the body. After consuming a meal high in carbohydrates, blood glucose increases swiftly as a result of the intestinal transporters' speedy action. The blood glucose that is absorbed in the intestines is subsequently distributed to every region of the body by the heart's pumping function.

All body cells can be reached by glucose in circulation, but it cannot enter them since accessing cells involves crossing a cell membrane, which glucose cannot accomplish on its own. Two proteins aid in the entry of circulatory glucose into cells. The first is referred to as a GLUT protein or glucose transporter. We should understand that the pancreas releases the hormone insulin into circulation to aid cells in absorbing glucose from the blood as the second factor.

CHAPTER 2

DISCOVERING GLUCOSE SPIKES and WHY ARE HARMFUL

12 EASY STEPS TO AVOID BLOOD SUGAR SPIKES

After eating, this happens when your blood sugar increases and then suddenly drops.

They may result in short-term fatigue and appetite. Type 2 diabetes may develop over time if your body is unable to adequately control blood sugar.

Diabetes is a growing public health issue. In reality, 25% of the 29 million Americans who have diabetes don't even realize they have.

Your blood arteries may stiffen and constrict as a result of blood sugar fluctuations, which increases your risk of having a heart attack or stroke.

Let's examine 12 easy steps you may take to avoid blood sugar spikes.

1. Get Low-Carb

Blood sugar levels to increase as a result of consuming carbohydrates. Carbohydrates are transformed into simple sugars when you ingest them. The bloodstream is subsequently filled with that glucose.

When your blood sugar levels rise, your pancreas releases the hormone insulin, which triggers your cells to start absorbing sugar from the blood. As a consequence, your blood sugar levels drop.

A low-carb diet has been found in several trials to help reduce blood sugar rises.

Additionally, low-carb diets may help with weight reduction, which helps lessen blood sugar rises. You may cut your carb consumption in many different ways, including by keeping track of them. Here is a how-to manual for the task.

2. **Consume less refined carbohydrates,** sometimes referred to as processed carbohydrates, such as sweets or refined grains. Refined carbs are often found in foods like table sugar, white bread, white rice, soda, candy, breakfast cereals, and desserts.

   Refined carbohydrates are devoid of almost all vitamins, minerals, fiber, and other nutrients. Because they are metabolized by the body so fast and readily, refined carbohydrates are considered to have a high glycemic index. As a result, blood sugar levels increase.

An increase in type 2 diabetes was linked to a diet heavy in carbohydrates with a high glycemic index, according to significant observational research including more than 91,000 women.

After consuming meals with a high glycemic index, your blood sugar may jump and then decrease, which may increase appetite, cause overeating, and result in weight gain.

Carbs have a variable glycemic index. It depends on a lot of factors, such as ripeness, what else you consume, and how the carbohydrates are prepared or cooked.

In general, whole-grain foods, along with the majority of fruits, non-starchy vegetables, and legumes, have a lower glycemic index.

3. Limit your sugar consumption.

The daily intake of added sugar in America is 22 teaspoons (88 grams). That is 350 calories. The majority of this comes from processed and prepared meals like candy, cookies, and sodas, while some of it is added as table sugar.

High-fructose corn syrup and sucrose are added sugars that you do not need nutritionally. In reality, they are merely empty calories. These simple sugars are extremely rapidly broken down by your body, which results in a very instantaneous rise in blood sugar.

Sugar consumption has been linked to the development of insulin resistance, according to studies. When this occurs, the body is unable to properly manage blood sugar because the cells do not react to the release of insulin as they should.

The US Food and Drug Administration (FDA) revised the requirements for food labeling in the US in 2016. Foods now need to list their added sugar content in grams and as a percentage of the daily recommended consumption. Sugar replacements may be used as an alternative to completely giving up sugar.

4. Maintain a healthy weight

Currently, it is estimated that two out of every three persons in the US are overweight or obese.

Obesity might make it more challenging for your body to utilize insulin and regulate blood sugar levels. This may result in blood sugar increases and an increased risk of type 2 diabetes.

There is a ton of data that connects obesity to insulin resistance and the onset of type 2 diabetes, while the exact mechanisms by which it occurs are still unknown.

On the other side, it has been shown that losing weight improves blood sugar regulation. In one research, 35 obese persons consumed 1,600 calories per day for 12 weeks and dropped an average of 14.5 pounds (6.6 kg). Their blood sugar levels decreased by 14% on average. Weight reduction was shown to reduce the risk of type 2 diabetes by 58% in another research of adults without diabetes.

5. Workout more

Exercise improves your cells' sensitivity to the insulin hormone, reducing blood sugar rises. Exercise also decreases blood sugar levels because muscle cells take up sugar from the circulation. Exercise has been demonstrated to reduce blood sugar peaks at any intensity, whether strong or moderate.

One research indicated that 27 individuals who engaged in either medium- or high-intensity exercise saw comparable benefits in blood sugar management. Exercise on an empty stomach or one that is already full may affect blood sugar regulation.

According to one research, exercising before breakfast successfully lowers blood sugar levels compared to exercising later. The increasing activity also aids in weight reduction, providing a double punch to blood sugar spike prevention.

6. Consume more fiber

The components of plant meals that your body is unable to digest make up fiber.

It is often split into two categories: soluble fiber and insoluble fiber.

Particularly soluble fiber may aid in reducing blood sugar increases.

When dissolved in water, it transforms into a gel-like substance that slows down the stomach's ability to absorb carbs. This produces a gradual rise and fall in blood sugar levels as opposed to a rush. Additionally, fiber might help you feel full, which can lessen your appetite and food consumption.

Soluble fiber comes from good sources like

- Oatmeal
- Nuts
- Legumes
- Several fruits, including blueberries, oranges, and apples
- several vegetables

7. Take extra water.

Lack of water intake might cause blood sugar to increase. When you are dehydrated, your body produces the hormone vasopressin. As a consequence, the body is prohibited from excreting additional sugar in your urine, and your kidneys are urged to retain fluid. Your liver also releases more sugar into the blood as a consequence of it.

A study of 3,615 people found that those who drank at least 34 ounces (about 1 liter) of water daily had a 21% reduced chance of getting high blood sugar than those who drank 16 ounces (473 ml) or less.

An increase in vasopressin levels in the blood was shown to be associated with an increase in insulin resistance and type 2 diabetes over a period of 12.6 years in long-term research, including 4,742 persons in Sweden. It's debatable how much water is ideal to consume. Basically, it depends on the person. You should always drink as soon as you feel thirsty, and you should drink more water in hot weather and when exercising. Instead of consuming sugary beverages or sodas, which can raise blood sugar levels, drink water.

8. Increase your consumption of vinegar.

Numerous health advantages of vinegar, especially apple cider vinegar, have been discovered.

It has been connected to improvements in blood sugar management, cholesterol reduction, and weight loss. Consuming vinegar may boost insulin responsiveness and lessen blood sugar increases, according to research.

In research, those who had just eaten a meal with 50 grams of carbohydrates discovered that vinegar drastically lowered their blood sugar levels. The research also discovered that blood sugar levels decreased with increasing vinegar strength.

Another research examined the impact of vinegar on blood sugar levels after carbohydrate consumption. It was discovered that vinegar raised insulin sensitivity from 19% to 34%. A food's glycemic index may be lowered by adding vinegar, which can help prevent blood sugar increases. According to Japanese research, eating pickled items with rice dramatically lowers the meal's glycemic index.

9. Get enough magnesium and chromium

According to studies, magnesium, and chromium are both capable of reducing blood sugar peaks.

Chromium

You require trace levels of the mineral chromium.

It is believed to improve how well insulin works. Helping the cells to absorb sugar from the blood may help regulate blood sugar rise.

In one tiny trial, 75 grams of white bread with or without additional chromium were given to 13 healthy males. After the meal, blood sugar dropped by roughly 20% as a consequence of the chromium supplementation.

Chromium dietary recommendations are available. Broccoli, egg yolks, shrimp, tomatoes, and Brazil nuts are examples of rich foods.

Magnesium

Another mineral that has been connected to blood sugar regulation is magnesium.

In research with 48 participants, half received lifestyle counseling alone while the other half also received a 600-mg magnesium supplement. In the group that received magnesium supplements, insulin sensitivity improved.

Another research examined the combined effects of chromium and magnesium supplementation on blood sugar. They discovered that taking both supplements together had a greater impact on insulin sensitivity than taking each supplement by itself. Rich food sources of magnesium include spinach, almonds, avocados, cashews, and peanuts.

10. Spice up your life a little.

Since ancient times, fenugreek and cinnamon have been utilized in traditional medicine. Both of these have been connected to blood sugar regulation.

Cinnamon

There is conflicting scientific data supporting the use of cinnamon to manage blood sugar.

In healthy people, cinnamon has been found to enhance insulin sensitivity and reduce blood sugar spikes after meals heavy in carbohydrates. Fourteen healthy participants were monitored in one of these trials.

In comparison to consuming the pudding alone, it was shown that consuming 6 grams of cinnamon together with 300 grams of rice pudding considerably lowered blood sugar surges.

Studies have also shown that cinnamon has no impact on blood sugar levels.

In a single analysis, 10 high-quality trials, including 577 diabetic patients, were examined. No discernible variation in blood sugar increases after individuals' use of cinnamon, according to the research.

Two varieties of cinnamon exist

- **Cassia:** Can be derived from a variety of Cinnamomum tree species. The majority of supermarkets carry this kind the most often.
- **Ceylon:** Specifically from the Cinnamomum verum tree in Ceylon. Although it costs more, it could have more antioxidants.

Coumarin, a compound found in cassia cinnamon, has the potential to be dangerous.

The acceptable daily intake of coumarin has been defined by the European Food Safety Authority (EFSA) at 0.045 mg per pound of body weight (0.1 mg/kg). For a 165-pound (75 kg) individual, this is equivalent to around half a teaspoon (1 gram) of Cassia cinnamon.

Fenugreek

The seeds of fenugreek are rich in soluble fiber, which is one of its qualities.

As a result, the digestion and absorption of carbohydrates are slowed, assisting in preventing blood sugar increases.

However, it seems that more than simply the seeds may help to lower blood sugar levels.

Two hours after eating, fenugreek dramatically lowered blood sugar levels, according to an analysis of 10 research.

Blood sugar peaks may be lessened with fenugreek. Although it may be added to meals, some individuals choose to take it as a supplement because of its strong flavor.

11. Attempt berberine

A molecule called berberine may be obtained from several plants.

It has been used for countless years in traditional Chinese medicine. Blood sugar regulation, weight loss, and cholesterol-lowering are a few of their applications. The liver produces less sugar when berberine is present, and it also improves insulin sensitivity. Even some medications intended to treat type 2 diabetes have been discovered to be as effective as it.

In one trial, 116 individuals with type 2 diabetes were given berberine or a placebo over a period of three months. After meals, berberine lowered blood sugar rises by 25%.

However, different research discovered that some participants who took berberine had adverse effects, including flatulence, diarrhea, and constipation. Although berberine seems to be rather safe, if you have any medical concerns or are taking any medications, see your doctor before using it.

12. Think about these lifestyle elements

You should also take into account these lifestyle variables that might alter blood sugar if you are serious about lowering your blood sugar spikes.

• Stress

Stress may result in a variety of health issues, such as headaches, high blood pressure, and anxiety.

Blood sugar levels have also been demonstrated to be impacted. Your body produces certain hormones when your level of stress increases. The fight-or-flight response is triggered, releasing sugary stored energy into your circulation. An increase in work-related stress was shown to be directly correlated with an increase in blood sugar levels in one research of 241 Italian employees.

Your blood sugar has been shown to improve from actively managing stress. Yoga poses have been shown in a study of nursing students to lessen stress, and blood sugar rises after meals.

• Sleep

Poor blood sugar regulation has been linked to both too little and too much sleep. Even one or two sleepless nights might have an impact on your blood sugar levels.

Sleeping too little, or for just four hours, raised insulin resistance and blood sugar levels, according to a study of nine healthy individuals.

Quality of sleep is just as important as quantity. According to research, the deepest stage of sleep (NREM) is crucial for maintaining blood sugar management.

● Alcohol

Alcoholic beverages often include a lot of extra sugar. For instance, mixed beverages and cocktails, which may include up to 30 grams of sugar per serving, fall under this category. Similar to added sugar in food, the sugar in alcoholic beverages will cause blood sugar to increase. Additionally, few alcoholic drinks provide much in the way of nutrition. Like added sugar, they are basically empty calories.

In addition, chronic excessive drinking might reduce insulin efficiency, which results in high blood sugar and, ultimately, type 2 diabetes. However, research indicates that regulated, moderate drinking may actually protect against type 2 diabetes development and improve blood sugar regulation. According to one research, consuming alcohol with meals in moderation may cut blood sugar rises by as much as 37%.

CHAPTER 3

GLUCOSE CURVE FLATTENING TECHNIQUES

A key marker of metabolic health is the amount of glucose that rises in your blood after eating and drinking. Following a meal, it is typical for your blood sugar to increase and then drop as your body absorbs the sugar from your blood to utilize for energy or to store. However, having consistently high blood glucose levels is bad for us.

According to studies, rather than monitoring calories, we should focus on flattening our post-meal glucose curves if we wish to control and maintain a healthy weight. You can eat more calories and burn more fat if your blood glucose curves are flatter compared to folks who eat fewer calories but don't put as much effort into doing so.

Your blood sugar curves will become flattered if you avoid blood sugar spikes.

Our time spent in fat-burning mode increases, and we experience fewer cravings and lower hunger when our blood glucose curves are flattened.

Blood glucose levels are maintained in a healthy range by the hormones insulin and glucagon working in tandem. Insulin triggers the cells to take up sugar as blood sugar levels rise, lowering blood sugar levels. Glucagon increases the release of glucose from the liver that has been stored when blood glucose levels fall too low. Together, they guarantee that cells have adequate energy to perform at all times.

Our bodies need glucose as an energy source, and we have mechanisms in place to handle and store it for later use. The main glycogen storage organs are the liver and muscles, and insulin helps us store roughly 15g of glycogen per kg of body weight (or about 1kg for a 70kg person). Insulin doesn't preferentially store energy anywhere, but 75% of the glucose transporters are in muscles, and 25% are in fat, and if we are eating the right amount, the energy stored in adipose tissue gets burned. The problem arises when we eat too much or eat high-GI foods because insulin also pushes glucose into adipose tissue. Additionally, fructose, which is metabolized by the liver and found in sugary meals, is transformed and stored as fat when there are extra calories as opposed to being converted to glucose (which is what occurs if you aren't overconsuming sugar or fructose).

Our insulin levels are persistently increased, and losing weight becomes much more difficult when blood glucose levels are consistently high. Reduced insulin levels are necessary for weight loss and always come first when blood glucose levels are reduced3. If we don't control our insulin levels, we go from fat-burning to fat-storage mode.

With the proper assistance, achieving blood sugar balance and reducing post-meal blood glucose rises may be simple and durable. The following resources can help maintain a healthy insulin and blood sugar response.

➢ **Eat Your Meals In The Proper Sequence:**

Calories from the four dietary categories, carbs (starch and sugar), protein, and healthy fats, all affect our blood sugar in very varied ways. We must consume the different food categories in a certain sequence in order to effectively regulate our post-meal blood sugar increases. The best strategy to reduce glucose spikes, according to a study, is to eat your veggies first, followed by your protein and fats, and then your carbs.

A sudden rise in blood glucose is brought on by the rapid breakdown of carbohydrates and sugars into glucose and its absorption into circulation. The sugar rise will be significantly greater if carbohydrates and sweets are ingested separately. Fat and protein also slow down the rate at which carbs leave the stomach because they take longer to digest than carbohydrates and delay gastric emptying. Vegetable fiber goes directly to the colon without being converted to glucose. Fiber also slows down digestion and decreases the availability of enzymes that convert carbohydrates into glucose; if the carbohydrates cannot be converted into glucose, their molecules are too big to be absorbed from the stomach into the blood. Due to the fact that fiber is not digested, it passes through the intestines as a viscous mesh, trapping more nutrients (such as lipids) and causing the production of hormones that prolong feelings of fullness. Additionally, it serves as food for the microbiota, which uses it to produce short-chain fatty acids that may reduce blood sugar levels and help us feel fuller for longer.

➤ With A Low Glycemic Index (Gi) Breakfast, You May Reduce Your Curves.

The Glycemic Index (GI) evaluates foods from 1-100 based on how rapidly they raise blood sugar levels after consumption. Foods with a low GI are broken down more gradually, which raises blood sugar gradually. High-GI meals, on the other hand, digest swiftly and raise blood sugar levels quickly.

You may start the day in "low GI" mode, sometimes referred to as a fat-burning mode, by eating a protein-rich breakfast. You will get long-lasting energy from this and have reduced between-meal hunger. Restricting carbs at breakfast is a straightforward method for preventing sharp spikes in blood sugar.

Your blood sugar reaction to breakfast will be healthier if you have a low GI breakfast in the morning, and your body will be better prepared to handle your next meal.

Therefore, even if you have a high GI lunch, if you begin your day in "low GI" mode, your blood sugar reaction will be less. The GI of one meal may affect the glycemic response to a later meal, a phenomenon known as the "second meal effect." The second meal effect helps with weight control in addition to a decreased postprandial (post-meal) glucose response.

➢ Adapt Your Carbs

When consumed in combination with fiber, protein, and lipids, sugars and carbohydrates may decrease how much and how fast your body absorbs glucose.

When consumed in isolation from other food categories, carbohydrates raise blood sugar levels, which causes us to feel momentarily satisfied but then rapidly need more food as levels increase and fall. High sugar consumption over time might impair hunger and fullness signals and increase cravings.

The glucose spikes that occur in reaction to carbohydrates and sweets are shortened by fiber, good fats, and protein. Due to the fact that they take longer to digest and have little effect on blood sugar, protein, healthy fats, and non-starchy veggies help us feel full for longer.

Simply include a green beginning or veggies with every meal, pair your snack with cheese or yogurt, or eat it with a handful of nuts and seeds to dress your carbohydrates.

➢ **After Your Main Meal, Indulge In Your Sweets.**

We get an immediate energy boost after eating anything sweet as the brain releases the feel-good chemical dopamine. Sucrose, which is composed of fructose and glucose molecules, is a component of sweet foods. Sugary meals produce a rise in both glucose and fructose levels.

However, fructose can only be stored as fat, whereas glucose may be stored in the liver and muscles as glycogen.

Compared to eating something sweet as a snack between meals and on an empty stomach, eating something sweet towards the conclusion of a meal will lessen the following glucose surge. This is due to the fact that although carbohydrates boost our blood sugar levels, their impact is lessened if we eat them together with vegetables, fat, and protein.

The time immediately after a meal is referred to as the postprandial stage, and this is when our metabolism is working hardest to break down nutrients and provide our tissues with vital metabolic fuels. Our insulin levels fall when we are not in the postprandial period, which helps us burn fat rather than retain it.

Your metabolism will want additional food as a result of snacking. The more meals you consume during the day, the more time your body will spend accumulating fat rather than burning it. To prevent an unhealthful blood sugar surge, it is preferable to eat a savory snack if you feel like one. Recent research suggests that eating bigger meals less often, as opposed to nibbling every few hours, may help us lose weight and boost metabolic flexibility.

➢ Exercise right after eating

The glucose curve after a meal may be flattened by going for a stroll. After eating, if we don't move about, our blood sugar levels will climb. Exercise causes the muscles to absorb blood glucose, reducing the blood glucose increase. After eating, we have up to 70 minutes to benefit from activity and flatten our glucose curve. Because muscles don't require insulin to absorb glucose while they are contracting, movement reduces our glucose surge without raising our insulin levels. The effect might be obtained with only a ten-minute stroll.

While exercising after a meal flattens the glucose curve more, exercising before a meal also helps minimize our spikes. Exercise after a meal helps curb appetites, stabilize moods, and prevent afternoon fatigue9.

Maintaining a stable blood sugar level prevents your cells from being overburdened with insulin, allowing your body to burn fat for energy in between meals and eventually leading to weight reduction.

You may lose weight without giving up the things you like by making little modifications to your eating habits, which also help your body function more effectively.

Try these methods to flatten your glucose curve if you want to control your blood sugar, become healthier, and reduce weight:

- Before every meal, have a modest salad or a dish of vegetables along with some healthy fats.
- Eat a savory breakfast as opposed to a sugary one.
- Never eat dessert or a sweet treat before or just after a meal.
- To get the benefits of fiber, choose whole fruit rather than juice.
- Eat the vegetables first, followed by the proteins, then the sweets and carbohydrates last throughout a meal.
- Never consume carbohydrates or sweets on an empty stomach.
- Never consume carbohydrates alone; instead, combine them with protein and wholesome fats.

- After every meal, take a 10-minute stroll. Any 10-minute workout that is done 70 minutes after eating will be beneficial.

CHAPTER 4

EAT YOUR MEAL IN THIS ORDER TO REDUCE BLOOD SUGAR SPIKE BY 75%

We understand if the concept of eating just meals that balance blood sugar makes you feel overwhelmed (or constrained). But there's more to it than simply what you're eating when it comes to preventing needless glucose surges. In fact, there is one method you may use without any dietary restrictions: Consume your food in a certain sequence.

For proper blood sugar regulation, eating your meals in sequence is ideal.

You may be wondering whether eating a meal in a certain sequence truly makes a difference. Let the research speak for itself, then: According to scientific research, consuming a meal's components in a certain sequence may lower the meal's glucose surge by 75%. "So you're consuming the same thing, but your body feels the effects considerably less.

The following is the optimal sequence:
- Vegetables first
- Fats and protein come next.
- Sugars and starches last.

Do you want to know how this seems in action? Imagine that you are enjoying a home-cooked lunch with a portion of nutritious salmon, spinach, and brown rice, as well as a piece of cake for dessert (we highly suggest one of these Mediterranean-diet-inspired sweet treats). The spinach should be consumed first, followed by the salmon, the rice, and the dessert.

On the other side, if you're dining out, I suggest the following blood sugar trick: Avoid devouring the free bread before a meal since doing so causes a significant glucose increase in the body. As a result, by the time they complete their main course, they are experiencing a severe glucose crash, feeling very hungry, and developing cravings. That's not to suggest you should completely avoid the bread basket; if you wait to have it with your protein, lipids, and veggies, your glucose reaction will be much more stable.

Speaking of vegetables, consider adding a high-quality greens powder with a rich dose of fiber, like mbg's organic veggies+, to your home-cooked meals if you want to give them even more blood-sugar-balancing punch. This USDA-certified organic supplement contains a variety of rare organic berries, vegetables, and herbs, pre-and probiotics, vegan-friendly digestive enzymes, and hard-to-find sea vegetables like kelp and chlorella. This special mixture has the ability to improve digestion and support stable blood sugar levels. So eating your vegetables first may aid in maintaining stable blood sugar levels, but adding organic vegetables on top can provide extra glucose-stabilizing advantages.

Remember that sugary beverages like sweetened tea might also have an impact on your blood sugar. Therefore, if you want to add a sweet beverage to your meal, be sure to save it as a treat and have it towards the end rather than earlier (this includes natural sweeteners too).

It's not necessary to restrict your strategic eating for blood sugar balance to a certain set of foods (although there are some blood-sugar-balancing foods worth noting). Because it works with any meal, eating your meal in a certain sequence might help you prevent a blood sugar surge. Additionally, it is simple to remember: Vegetables come first, followed by protein and fats, and then carbs and sweets.

By adopting simple dietary changes, such as following a low-carb, high-fiber diet and staying away from added sugars and processed carbs, you may be able to reduce blood sugar spikes.

Beyond aiding in blood sugar regulation, frequent exercise, keeping a healthy weight, and drinking lots of water may all be beneficial to your health.

Having said that, consult your doctor before making any dietary changes if you have any medical concerns or are taking any drugs.

Making these simple dietary and lifestyle adjustments is usually a smart strategy to reduce your risk of type 2 diabetes or insulin resistance.

CHAPTER 5

WHEN IS A NORMAL GLUCOSE LEVEL

High And Low Glucose Level Risk

Normal Levels of Blood Glucose

The best blood glucose levels for an individual depend on their age, the drugs they take, the stage and duration of their diabetes, as well as any other illnesses that may affect blood sugar.

There are some basic suggestions to remember, even though you should always discuss your goal blood glucose levels with your healthcare provider:

- **Fasting blood glucose (between meals):** Between meals, a person's fasting blood sugar should range between 70 and 100 mg/dL.

- **Preprandial glucose (before a meal):** Blood sugar levels before eating should range from 80 to 130 milligrams per deciliter (mg/dL) in adults who are not pregnant, from less than 95 mg/dL in women who have gestational diabetes, and from 70 to 95 mg/dL in women who already have type 1 or type 2 diabetes.

- **Postprandial glucose (1-2 hours after a meal):** The goal for individuals who are not pregnant with postprandial glucose (one to two hours after a meal) is fewer than 180 mg/dL. The goal for those with gestational diabetes is less than 140 mg/dL one hour after eating and fewer than 120 mg/dL two hours after eating. One hour after a meal, pregnant women with type 1 or type 2 diabetes should have levels between 110 and 140 mg/dL, and two hours after a meal, they should be between 100 and 120 mg/dL.

- **Before engaging in any exercise:** Exercise may deplete energy and result in low blood sugar. Pre-exercise blood sugar levels should generally fall between 126 mg/dL to 180 mg/dL.

- **After physical activity:** If your blood sugar level is below 100 mg/dL after exercise, consider consuming 15 to 20 grams of carbohydrates to boost it. If your blood sugar measurement is still below 100 mg/dL after 15 minutes, consume another serving of 15 grams of carbohydrates. In order to reach the 100 mg/dL minimum level, repeat this procedure every 15 minutes. 17 It is known as the 15-15 rule.

What Factors Can Affect Glucose Levels?

In addition to food, activity, and how well your body generates and utilizes insulin, several additional aspects, including

- Sleep deprivation
- Caffeine intake
- Angst levels
- Becoming sunburnt
- Leaving out food
- Not drinking enough water.
- The time of day, since controlling blood sugar levels later, appears to be more challenging for some ailments, such as gum disease.

What Is the A1C Test?

A blood test called the A1C, also known as the HbA1C, hemoglobin A1C, glycated hemoglobin, or glycosylated hemoglobin test, aids in the monitoring and diagnosis of diabetes. This examination evaluates your blood sugar levels on average over the previous two to three months.

High Glucose Risks

Type 1 and type 2 diabetes are the two varieties. The immune system targets and kills the pancreatic cells that produce insulin in type 1 diabetes. Your body cannot produce enough insulin or utilize it efficiently if you have type 2 diabetes. The most prevalent kind of diabetes is type 2.

Hyperglycemia may result from diabetes. Hyperglycemia is indicated by blood glucose levels that are more than 180 mg/dL two hours after eating or higher than 130 mg/dL when fasting. Hyperglycemia is defined as blood glucose levels that are more than 200 mg/dL at any moment.

Too high blood sugar levels can:

- Increase the frequency of urination as the kidneys attempt to excrete more blood glucose via urine.
- Make someone thirstier.
- Heart disease, heart attacks, and stroke are possibly brought on by damage to blood arteries throughout your body.
- Lead to visual haziness, unhealing wounds, skin infections, and vaginal yeast infections.

- Increase the likelihood of developing diabetic retinopathy, an eye disease.

Diabetic ketoacidosis is a potentially fatal illness that may arise from high blood sugar levels (DKA). When there is insufficient insulin in the body, body fat is burned as energy instead of blood sugar. When ketones are produced, your blood may become acidic if their levels are high. Type 1 diabetes is more likely to have this disease.

A medical emergency is DKA. Extreme mouth dryness, nausea, vomiting, shortness of breath, and fruity breath are some of the signs of DKA.

Risks of Low Glucose

Low blood sugar is defined as having blood glucose levels below 70 mg/dL. Severe low blood sugar is defined as a value below 54 mg/dL. One or two times each week, people with diabetes, particularly those with type 1 diabetes, may have low blood sugar.

While they are sleeping, some people may have low blood sugar. If you consume alcohol, use excessive insulin, or have had a very busy day, this might occur.

The following are examples of hypoglycemia symptoms and risks:

- Rapid heart rate
- Sweating and trembling
- Nervousness
- Feeling perplexed
- Feeling peckish
- Dizziness

Significantly low blood sugar might cause more significant problems, such as extreme fatigue, trouble moving, and blurred vision. Additionally, it may cause convulsions or even unconsciousness.

When To Visit A Physician

If you encounter signs of hyperglycemia or hypoglycemia, get in touch with your healthcare professional. If you are experiencing trouble managing your blood sugar levels, it is extremely vital to see your doctor since this might indicate more significant, perhaps life-threatening, health issues.

CHAPTER 6

TROUBLESHOOTING GLUCOSE TRANSFORMATION

Common Inquiries And Practical Responses/Solutions

High Glucose: What Does It Mean?

Hyperglycemia, often known as high blood sugar, occurs when the body either produces insufficient amounts of the hormone insulin or cannot adequately use it to transport glucose into cells for use as fuel.

Where Does The Body Store Glucose?

Extra glucose is turned into a kind of energy called glycogen and stored in your muscles and liver until your body has utilized all of it for energy.

How Can You Reduce Your Blood Sugar Levels?

You may reduce high blood sugar levels in a number of ways, including via exercise, dietary changes, and the use of diabetic medications. Consult your healthcare practitioner to learn which tactics will benefit you the most.

What Brings About Hypoglycemia?

There are several potential reasons. It may happen to diabetics when they don't eat enough or regularly enough, when they exercise or just after, or when they take too much insulin or medicine. It may be brought on by excessive alcohol consumption, some blood sugar-lowering drugs, certain diseases, hormone shortages, or an excess of insulin in people without diabetes.

How Is Hypoglycemia Managed?

In moderate situations, blood sugar may be stabilized using glucose tablets or high-sugar meals or beverages every 15 minutes as necessary. Prescription medications that include the hormone glucagon, which causes the release of glucose from storage in extreme circumstances (including loss of consciousness in diabetics), may be utilized. If blood sugar levels do not rise, immediate medical care is required.

What Signs Or Symptoms Indicate Hypoglycemia?

Shaking, a rapid pulse, perspiration, exhaustion, worry, and hunger are typical symptoms. An extremely low blood sugar level may cause symptoms including disorientation, blurred vision, behavioral abnormalities, slurred speech, seizures, or loss of consciousness.

How Is Hypoglycemia Detected?

If a diabetic's blood sugar falls below 70 mg/dL, they may use their blood glucose meter to check. People without diabetes who have hypoglycemia symptoms, particularly if they are persistent, should see a doctor who can order blood tests, enquire about their medical history, and do a physical examination in an effort to identify the underlying cause of the hypoglycemia.

CONCLUSION

Diabetes patients often suffer from blood sugar rises shortly after eating. Hyperglycemia is the medical term for high blood sugar. Typically, using insulin, medicines, or dietary changes may reduce these increases.

Complications may arise when a person's blood sugar rises are not controlled. Some of these might endanger your life.

By working with their doctor to receive the proper diabetic medication and dosage and practicing a preventative lifestyle that includes a suitable diet and enough exercise, a person may avoid problems.

Even those without diabetes sometimes suffer from blood sugar increases. This may occur as a consequence of stress, a physical injury, or an illness.

Because glucose is the primary energy source for our cells, it is crucial for our bodies to operate correctly. Numerous health issues may arise when the quantity of glucose in our blood is either too high or too low.

If neglected, it may have an impact on a number of bodily organs, including the kidneys and the eyes. As a result, if you have diabetes, work with your doctor to develop the best strategy for maintaining a normal blood sugar level.

Knowing your blood glucose levels is essential since readings that are either too high or too low might be harmful to your general health. The best course of action is to develop a treatment plan with your healthcare physician since optimum blood sugar levels might differ significantly from person to person. You may decide how to manage your levels most effectively together.

An essential step in avoiding diabetic complications is controlling blood sugar levels. Blood sugar levels that remain within a modest range might show that a therapy is effective.

At the beginning of therapy, a doctor will establish objectives because each patient's requirements are unique. As the course of therapy develops, they could modify these goals. Anyone who is worried about their blood sugar levels should contact a doctor.